BREAST PTOSIS:

THE PHENOMENON OF BREAST SAGGING

BY

STEPHANIE W. CROOKS

Table of Contents

Introduction

Without or with firm breasts, every lady is stunning. But occasionally you may ponder the genuine reason behind your twins' sagging. Is it a result of a health problem or is it natural? Knowing more about your body is never a bad thing, which is why it's best you understand the reason why your breasts are sagging. Many women cope with this problem, which is rather frequent. Thankfully, there are some situations where sagging can be reversed; in other situations, you can't truly control it.

Unfortunately, some breast sagging is unavoidable—I am sorry to break the bad news. Collagen, the connective tissue under the skin, loses its elasticity as a result of pregnancy, breastfeeding, and adding birthdays, leaving your breast more deflated than firm. Genetics may play a role in sag as well. You might be susceptible to one if your mother had a pair that sagged.

The truth is that several breast activities that might seem unrelated to sag can in fact cause it; as a result, your breasts will benefit if you avoid them. You might wish to stop any habit connected to a flaccid pair—like these—given that a recent UCLA study discovered that breast tissue ages two to three years faster than the rest of your body.

Chapter 1

What Are Breasts?

Both male and female sexual anatomy include breasts. Breasts are both functional (for lactation) and sexual organs in females (bringing pleasure). The function of male breasts is nonexistent. Nipples and areolae are among the breast anatomy that can be seen.

The breast is a vital organ in a human. It is an organ found protruding on the chest of the woman filled with breast milk. It can appear in different shapes and sizes.

Generally, every maturing and matured female has a pair of breasts and they serve the same purpose despite the variations. A woman's breasts typically develop during the majority of her life. It has various stages in between, starts before birth, and finishes at menopause.

Each woman will experience the stages at a different time because they correspond with her life's phases. For those who are transitioning their gender, these stages will alter as well. One person to the next will have very different breast sizes. In any event, it's critical to understand typical development so that you can identify any potential problems at an early stage.

Developing Breasts

The development of the breast is one of the earlier signs of puberty in girls. Girls may experience both exhilaration and fear as they adjust to their changing bodies throughout this time. At puberty, the ovaries release hormones that are responsible for breast development.

These hormones allow fat to build up, which increases the size of your breast

What Transpires When The Breast Grows?

Breast bud development, which is the earliest stage of breast growth, is characterized by a modest swelling under the nipple.

During the early stages of breast development, they can be extremely sensitive and painful. As your skin stretches, it could itch as well. An initial bra purchase might lessen discomfort and safeguard new breast growth. Skin stretch marks could develop if the breasts expand quickly.

With time, these will diminish.

With the girl's body fat rising during adolescence, the breasts will continue to develop. They expand and enlarge in size. The nipple may develop an erect or protruding appearance, and the areola (the region surrounding it) may get darker and larger. It is typical for one breast to develop more quickly than the other. Even so, many adult women discover that their breasts are only very little difference in size with time. Everything about this is normal.

Do Breasts Hurt As They Develop?

If so, why? Yes, when breasts develop, they can hurt. Estrogen and progesterone cause the breasts to enlarge. These hormone levels rise as you approach puberty. Under the stimulus of these hormones, your breasts start to develop. The menstrual cycle, pregnancy, lactation, and menopause can cause changes in hormone levels. The amount of fluid in your breasts changes as a result of hormones. Your breasts might feel more sensitive or uncomfortable as a result of this.

Around the time of her menstrual cycle, a young woman's breasts may pain if she has begun her period. These pains, which are brought on by hormonal fluctuations, are a typical aspect of the menstrual cycle.

How Long Does Breast Development Take?

Between the ages of 8 and 13, breast growth typically starts. Typically, a girl's breasts are fully formed by the age of 17 or 18, however, they can continue to develop into their early 20

Chapter 2

The Meaning of Sagging/Saggy Breast

The issue of the saggy or sagging breast has caused a lot of trauma to the females who are affected. S Like other parts of your body, the breasts will change with time. The nipple may point downward, the top of the breast may not be as full as it once was, and your breasts may appear to sit lower o the chest. The severity of breast ptosis is measured by the position of the nipple with the fold of the breast. When the nipple sits above the line of the fold, it is considered normal. When the nipple is even with the fold, it is described as first-degree ptosis. Second-degree ptosis is when the nipple is below the fold, and third-degree ptosis is seen when the nipple is pointing downwards.

At puberty, the young female starts to develop and feel the accumulation of fats around the chest region. This growth continues until the breast is fully formed.

The formed breast remains firm with the nipple pointing upwards. At this point, the breast is firm and standing. Unfortunately, with time, the breast will start to expand and gradually become saggy. Sagging of the breast is caused by many factors which include the following;

Aging

As people age, their bodies naturally produce fewer reproductive hormones, which can affect how the breasts look and feel.

Everyone is affected differently by aging. Age-related breast changes are mostly harmless and are a normal aspect of growing older.

Low estrogen levels and altered skin elasticity cause these alterations in the breasts. The risk of acquiring growths like fibroids, cysts, and cancer, all of which can alter the appearance of the breasts, also rises with age.

Gravitational pull

The force of gravity is the force that acts downwards. It tends to pull down objects downwards. The gravitational force works in proportionality to weight.

According to research, big breasts tend to fall more easily than smaller breasts due to the effect of gravitational pull on them. The bigger breasts will experience the force of gravity faster than the smaller breasts. This assertion is however opposed by some Biologists who practically believe that the force of gravity has no observable effects on the breast. The regular use of a fitted bra will go a long way in preventing the sagging of the breast by the gravitational pull or force.

Hormone Changes

Hormones regulate all the activities of the body. Different activities take place in the body and as such there are different hormones present in the body too.

The development of breasts at puberty by the female child is influenced by the action of estrogen. Estrogen is the hormone produced by the ovaries and its effects lead to the development of breasts in females. The more estrogen is produced in the body, the bigger the breast becomes, and vice versa.

Over time, estrogen levels reduce, which leads to a loss of gland tissue in the breast. Together with the changes in the elasticity of the skin, this may cause the breasts to get reduced than before.

The appearance of the nipple may be affected too. Sagging of the breast can be given different possible meanings. Scientifically, it is called Breast Ptosis.

The weight gain/loss

As a lady adds in weight or gains weight, no part of the body is left behind. Every part including the breast adds simultaneously. As you put on weight, your breast's fatty tissue increases, just like it does throughout the rest of your body. The connective tissue and ligaments that hold the breast to the chest are put under additional stress and pressure as a result of the breast area becoming heavier and larger. The fatty tissue in the breast shrinks away as you then shed the excess weight, but the stretched-out supporting ligaments beneath do not get tighter.

Overall, weight loss causes the breast envelope to deflate noticeably, and an inelastic pocket of extra surface skin appears in the breasts. This "sagging" can sometimes be seen with the naked eye and contributes to some emotional disturbance.

Smoking

One of the most crucial proteins in our bodies, collagen is in charge of keeping our skin elastic. As you get older, your reserves start to run out, but if you smoke, your production is slowed down eve more quickly, which causes sagging breasts.

Smoking is a significant contributor to breast sagging, or ptosis, as it damages the elastin protein that gives skin support and a more youthful appearance. Smokers truly do incur the danger of developing a prematurely saggy bust since both the essential components of elastin and collagen are under attack.

However, there is another, less evident explanation behind smokers' sagging breasts. It is commonly known that nicotine suppresses appetite and raises metabolic rate, which causes the body to burn calories more quickly

Multiple pregnancies

Women who have had multiple pregnancies are likely to experience breast ptosis. When a woman gets pregnant, the breast gets fuller and stretched. The breast gets fuller because certain hormonal changes are taking place in the breast thereby preparing the breast for the task of breastfeeding ahead. The breast continues to be full and in shape after childbirth but on weaning the child, the breast cannot go back to its original shape and by then the hormone for milk secretion must have been inactivated. Stretching of the ligaments in the breast over time. These ligaments are called "Cooper's ligaments"

Posture

Some scientists have concluded that most sagging breasts are a result of the body posture of the individual. Hunched or bent back posture can force the breast to stand on its own. The body ought to support the breast. A breast that stands on its own is likely to lose the elasticity of the ligament faster, thereby causing the breast to sag.

Excessive Sunburn

Sunburn affects the elasticity of the skin generally. Because of the skin damage caused by UV rays and the lack of elasticity, sunburn can also result in sagging breast. An exposed breast to the sun is likely to lose elasticity faster.

Regular exposure of the breast and other body parts to the sun will lead to sunburn which in turn affects the elasticity of the skin on these parts of the body. Women who are exposed to sunburn will have saggy breasts.

Menopause

Your estrogen levels drastically decrease as menopause approaches. Breast glandular tissue diminishes when your milk system begins to shut down. This results in them losing density and increasing fat, which can cause sagging. Additionally, one might see that the breasts are not as full as they once were and that their size has changed.

Chapter 3

Preventive measures/treatment of sagging breast

Aging comes naturally and there is absolutely nothing anyone can do about it. Apart from aging, several other factors lead to the sagging of the breast. The possible ways of preventing sagging of the breast and the treatment of the sagging breast are listed below;

Watch your weight

Weight fluctuations are not small weight gain or loss; they do not increase the risk of early breast drooping. But keep in mind that drastic weight changes will unquestionably result in early breast sagging. In actuality, as we grow older, our metabolism slows down, putting us at risk for drastic weight fluctuations brought on by aging. As a result, it's crucial that we work to keep our weight consistent.

Maintaining a stable, healthy weight is all that's necessary. Your breasts will become firmer and less likely to sag as a result of this.

Avoid Smoking/Quit Smoking Habit

There are several health issues that smoking and nicotine consumption can cause, some of which are fatal, like lung cancer. However, as we just said, smoking's toxins and nicotine itself can cause sagging breasts by destroying the elasticity in your skin. Therefore, quitting smoking is a straightforward strategy o maintain this crucial protein, which is in charge of maintaining the skin's elasticity throughout your body.

Avoid Sunburn by Using Sunscreen

Try to establish a daily routine of applying sunscreen. Ultraviolet (UV) rays can harm your skin, as we already discussed. Reduced skin collagen is one of the effects of UV radiation that frequently occurs. As early as your 20s, collagen production starts to slow down. The danger of premature aging in your skin and therefore your breasts increases if you are exposed to the sun for extended periods, such as if you frequently lie in indoor tanning beds. So that your skin is protected from the sun, we advise applying sunscreen.

Breast massages

Anecdotal research suggests that massaging your breasts may boost blood flow and encourage collagen formation, which may offer some lift by tightening muscles and encouraging tissue growth.

Use the following techniques to massage your breasts:

* Place one hand on top of the opposite breast;

* Gently squeeze the area;

* Gradually move your hand down the top of your breast; * Work your hand around the outside, under, and inner part of your breast using the same pumping motion;

* Alternate between squeezing and pumping with gentle fingertip circles.

Balance your Diet

Try to eat a well-balanced, healthy diet to nourish your skin and keep it that way for many years to come.

Keeping your weight at the right level for your body type is also crucial. When you are overweight, your skin tissue is under stress, and your breasts may gain weight as a result, which could cause sagging. Healthy lifestyle choices are essential in addition to a healthy diet. Both your skin and your general health are negatively impacted by tobacco use. It can be one of the contributing factors to sagging breasts.

 Make sure you stay hydrated by drinking enough water throughout the day. Drinking enough water will keep your skin robust and enhance your general health because it powers everything in your body.

Engage in Exercises

Breast tissue cannot be firmed up with exercising since it lacks muscle. To improve the overall appearance of your chest, you might exercise the muscles and fibrous connective tissue that are located beneath the breasts.

The chest region can benefit from a variety of exercises to strengthen muscles and correct posture. You might try the following common exercises: bench press, arm curls, and pushups in the pool.

Maintain a good posture

When the breasts hang by their weight due to poor posture, such as a hunched or bowed back, extra pressure and tension are placed on the breast tissue, which exacerbates sagging.

On the other hand, maintaining good posture entails instructing your body to adopt positions during movement that put the least amount of stress on the muscles and ligaments that provide support.

Good posture helps to appropriately distribute your body's weight and prevents sagging by keeping your back straight and shoulders back.

Wear fitted bra

This is particularly true with exercises like jogging. Breast mobility can be reduced by using a sports bra with lots of support (molded cups). More research is required, although one study indicates that breast motion from exercise causes stretching and sagging.

According to the same study, wearing a bra is not always necessary to prevent breast sagging when you are not working out. In fact, wearing the incorrect bra size can be worse for you than going without one.

Fruits to make your Breast Firmer and Perkier

Breasts change as you age, yet there are a few straightforward ways you reduce the process. The changes that take place in the breasts are inevitable.

Breasts require around five years to develop and will go through a host of changes over the years.

You might see they become tighter and full at specific times and afterward flatten somewhat at different times.

As your breasts age, they will likewise begin to sag, because of gravity, hormonal changes, and breastfeeding.

"As we age, skin loosens up and sags, so that is the reason there's that hang and they hang down lower, regardless of whether they're not that enormous," says Dr. Hazen. "Individuals consider big breasts dropping and smaller ones will sag in the long run, as well."

There are basic ways of keeping your breasts from falling and it doesn't need to undergo surgery.

Here we uncover five food varieties that can assist with keeping your bosoms firm:

1. Oranges

Oranges are wealthy in antioxidant beta-carotene that shields your breast cells from damage. They are likewise plentiful in calcium and vitamin B6 boosts and enhance the improvement of breasts.

2. Green vegetables

Green veggies such as spinach, broccoli, and kale are rich in phytoestrogens that are known to advance and promote breast tissue.

3. Pomegranate

Pomegranate has high antioxidant content that assists in cell regeneration and shields from untimely maturing. Pomegranate likewise diminishes the risk of cancer growth and helps in breast firming.

4. Soy

Soy is rich in isoflavones, soy items give bigger breast tissue. Besides, they additionally have a few estrogen-like supplements that promote breast improvement.

5. Strawberries

Rich in phytoestrogen and ellagic acid that make the breast skin spotless, smooth and tight.

Seven meals can help you tighten sagging breasts.

Here are some home remedies to firm up sagging breasts as well as seven meals that medical professionals recommend to help you do it.

1. Lentils

You can tighten your breasts by eating meals high in protein like lentils, dairy products, and eggs.

2. Beans

Beans are a good source of fiber and, by preserving the development of healthy tissue, they help to prevent breast sagging during pregnancy and due to advancing age.

3. Turmeric

In particular, following nursing, turmeric's anti-inflammatory qualities maintain healthy, smooth blood flow in the breasts and prevent sagging breasts.

4. Plum

Blueberries, plums, and peaches are all sources of antioxidants that fight aging and cancer. In addition to maintaining blood arteries open, these antioxidants help support smooth blood flow. The good blood flow will ensure that your bust stays fuller and firmer.

5. Nuts and seeds

Pumpkin, sunflower, flax, and anise seeds tend to increase estrogen levels naturally in the body, which helps to keep firm breasts. Along with seeds, nuts are beneficial for your breast size as they are a fantastic source of protein and fat.

6. Cruciferous vegetables

Broccoli, cabbage, and cauliflower are examples of cruciferous vegetables that contain phytoestrogens, which act like estrogen and support healthy breasts. No of the situation, keep in mind that you should consume green leafy vegetables every day.

7. Oily fish

Omega-3 fatty acids can be found in abundance in salmon, sardines, tuna, and other fatty fish. They can help repair the damage caused by free radicals, which makes them effective for elevating sagging breasts. In fact, studies on various shellfish have found that they raise sex hormone levels and promote the growth of breast tissue.

Chapter 4

Reducing the Breast Size

Throughout a woman's life, her breasts develop. Some women could view larger breasts as a healing tool. However, large breasts can be accompanied by a number of problems, including neck and back pain.

The fat and glandular tissue in the bosoms are connected by chemical receptors. The oily tissue that makes up the bosom is called fat tissue, but the glandular tissue, sometimes known as the "bosom tissue," is responsible for producing milk. These tissues may eventually expand and the bosoms may become larger as a result of hormonal changes in the body. Various factors can also influence one another. These comprise:

- Pregnancy
- Corpulence medicine
- Inheritable traits

Seven remedies that you can do at home

A medical procedure to reduce breast size is chosen by some women to avoid discomfort and increase portability. However, you can experiment with less invasive methods at home to reduce breast size. Before using any of these home remedies, consult your PCP.

1. Work-out

Normal activity can help with chest fat loss and build up the muscles under the breasts to reduce their size.

Focusing on cardio and intense focus exercises will help you lose weight more quickly and address pain locations because the breasts are partially made of fat.

Strenuous exercises, including step climbing, cycling, and power walking, can speed up digestion and help you reduce your overall muscle-to-fat ratio.

Pushups are one exercise that can condition the chest and alter the appearance of breasts. Pushups can tighten and tone your chest muscles, which will help to reduce your chest's overall size. However, just building your strength and doing specific exercises won't reduce your bust size. A few activities can make the bosoms appear larger without cardio or a full-body workout.

At least four times a week, 30 minutes of practice is advised.

2. Diet

Your body's ability to accumulate fat is influenced by the foods you eat. By and large, a high muscle-to-fat ratio can increase bust size.

Maintaining a balance between exercise and a healthy eating plan will help you lose weight and shrink your bust.

Consuming more calories than you burn off causes you to gain weight and develops your breasts.

Foods that help you burn fat in addition to your regular workout routine include lean meats, seafood, natural goods, and veggies. You can lose weight more quickly by consuming fewer processed food options and sweets.

3. Green tea

Another common remedy for promoting weight loss is green tea. Green tea has a variety of cell reinforcements and can aid in the digestion of fats and calories. Your breast size will shrink thanks to this reduced fat development. Throughout the day, drinking green tea might also help you feel more energized.

4. Ginger

Ginger has similar benefits to green tea in terms of boosting digestion and consuming excess body fat. Nutritionists advise drinking it as a tea three times per day to boost weight loss effects and speed up digestion, though you can add it to meals as a natural ingredient.

5. Flaxseed

A few unsaturated fats, particularly omega-3 unsaturated fats, are important for the function of the brain, lowering heart rate, and controlling chemical production. This is crucial for breast reduction because a chemical imbalance might trigger growth.

Unfortunately, our bodies only typically provide a small amount of the nutrients we need to thrive. We have to consume food types rich in these ingredients to obtain them. Omega-3 unsaturated fats are found in abundance in flax seeds, fish, and salmon. As a final result, it can help reduce breast size and help direct estrogen levels. It also has a reputation for affecting systems relating to your stomach.

Flax seed can be consumed with water or added to a variety of foods. Additionally, your local health food store may have ground flaxseed egg substitutes and non-dairy flaxseed milk.

6. Egg whites

By improving your complexion, you can also reduce the size of your breasts. After some time, breastfeeding, maturing, and weight loss may cause the breast to hang. This may sometimes give the impression that the breasts are larger than they actually are. To restore flexibility to your breast skin, try wearing an egg white veil.

Apply a froth created by beating two egg whites to your breasts. After 30 minutes, leave the cover in place and wash it off with warm water. You may see a recognizable firming of your skin as it dries. Nevertheless, as the egg whites break off or wash away, this is transient.

(7) Clothes

In the unlikely event that conventional treatments fail to help you, wearing well-fitting clothing may be an option to hide your breasts. Spend money on a bra that fits properly and supports and includes the breasts. The neck sections of your shirt should also be checked since they can draw attention away from your bust.

Chapter 5

Myths about Breast Sagging that's to be Abolished

First, a couple of truths: We'd all love to have perky breasts our whole lives, but sagging is just a part of life. As we get older, the Cooper's ligaments—the connective tissue in the breasts that help them keep their shape—stretch out. "Also, breasts gradually change from having more breast tissue to having more fat, and this can make them appear less perky and even deflated looking," says Anne Taylor, chair of the public education committee for the American Society of Plastic Surgeons and an adjunct associate professor in the department of plastic surgery at Ohio State University.

Many women will do just about anything they can to delay or even prevent sagging. But to do that properly, you need to get the sag story straight. Here, the top misconceptions about what makes the girls hang low:

Myth #1: Breastfeeding can cause sagging.

Not true. According to a 2008 study in the *Aesthetic Surgery Journal*, breastfeeding is not a risk factor for breast ptosis (another word for sagging). Actually, the pregnancy itself is probably the bigger culprit, says Mary Jane Minkin, MD, a clinical professor of obstetrics and gynecology at Yale University School of Medicine. " Breasts increase in size with pregnancy and stay enlarged with breastfeeding, but they then slowly shrink back down once a woman is done nursing," she says. "That weight loss and deflation of the breasts can make them sag."

Myth #2: Certain exercises can keep your breasts from sagging. Breasts don't contain muscle, so there aren't any exercises you can do to specifically target them. But Judy Blume didn't have it all wrong: Doing exercises for the chest muscles, specifically the pectoralis major muscle located directly underneath the breasts, can help elevate the breasts and give them a perkier appearance, says Deborah Axelrod, MD, medical director of clinical breast services and breast programs of New York University Langone Medical Center.

There's no data that shows that certain bras such as push-up bras prevent sagging, or that any particular kind of bra can cause sagging, says Minkin. Also, while wearing a bra to bed is totally fine for comfort, don't expect that nighttime support to keep your girls in perfect shape. Again, there's no proof that doing so will help prevent sagging. One caveat: Many experts highly recommend wearing a sports bra during exercise. "The constant pull of gravity and the bouncing and movement during running can stretch the breast tissue and possibly lead to sagging, so hold them up with a supportive bra," suggests Taylor. "Some sports bras are like body armor—they hold the breasts so well there is no movement at all."

Myth #3: Small breasts don't sag.

Even small breasts are subject to gravity—just not as much. "It is true that in general small breasts do sag a bit less than larger ones because there's less tissue pulling down," says Minkin. Adds Axelrod, "Whether or not your breasts sag depends on the ratio of breast tissue to fat.

In other words, if you have a high breast density—meaning there's more breast tissue compared to fat—your breasts will be less likely to droop than if you have a low breast density, with more fat than breast tissue. (Looking for ways to get in more exercise but you're seriously short on time? Check out super-effective workout DVD.)

Myth #4: There's nothing you can do to prevent sagging.

While sagging is inevitable for many women, you can take steps to at least minimize it. For instance, the study in the *Aesthetic Surgery Journal* found that a high BMI and a history of smoking were risk factors for breast sagging. Also, avoid yo-yo dieting. "If a woman gains a lot of weight, her breasts will stretch out just as the rest of her skin will," says Minkin. "However, if she then loses that weight, she'll be left with the extra skin, which just sags because it no longer has all that tissue holding it up. Always maintaining a healthy weight will likely help."

Myth #5: Exercise can tone the breasts

Some women think that toning up the chest is the way to prevent sagging. To be clear with the facts, breasts don't have muscles, so there is no way of firming them up with spot exercises. However, beneath your breast tissue are muscles which you can work on. So to put it more correctly, you simply tone your chest muscles and not your breasts. You can tone your Cooper's ligaments, which run along your chest, to make your breasts look perkier.

Myths #6: Wearing a bra 24/7 prevents breast sagging.

Some women believed that wearing their bra all the time prevents the dreaded ptosis (the medical term for breast sagging). This is actually no truth to this because just like anything in your body, your breasts eventually succumb to the ravages of aging. In fact, one research even said that wearing a bra can cause breast sagging because it weakens the muscles that hold up the breast. To some extent this might be right however never forgo proper support when doing strenuous exercises.

Myths #7 Your lifestyle doesn't have any bearing in breast sagging.

In insipid ways, your lifestyle choices can have a profound effect on the amount of sagging your breast face. Smoking, crash diets, and sun bathing can worsen the degree of breast sagging aside from the deterioration of the natural support and gravitational pull.

Smoking ages the skin because it hampers proper blood circulation which is necessary for nourishing the skin. Crash diets on the other hand lead to weight fluctuation, which we discussed about earlier. Sun bathing, even with the strongest sunscreen can also break down collagen which is the building block of your skin.

9 798355 799694